Health through Move, Relaxation and nutrition

How I changed my life in a positive way

Angelika Doerenberg

Born in 1966

Shiatsu practitioner since 2002 and yoga teacher since 2007

Self-experience and further education since 1990 in:

- Spinal exercises / back training
- yoga
- Qi Gong
- Autogenic training
- Brain Gym - Integration of the right and left brain hemispher es
- Chakra teaching
- Coping with stress through exercise and relaxation
- Feldenkrais
- Relaxation foot reflexology massage
- Shiatsu, basic craniosacral technique

Table of Contents

Prologue: How it all began

Already at a young age I was looking and asked myself the question: "Where is my place in life?", "What gives my life a meaning?"

I gradually found my way through meditation weekends, conversations and "desert days" that I attended in a monastery. Topics included situations from previous life, which I questioned using various methods. In addition to the conversations, there was, for example, the opportunity to paint intuitively and then interpret the pictures. Fantasy journeys or eutonia were also popular, in which I learned to feel into my body.

That's how I discovered spinal gymnastics in order to create a balance to my daily sitting. Then I wanted to create a balance not only for my body, but also for my soul and my spirit. That's how I got into yoga.

While attending yoga classes regularly, I realized that this philosophy will be my life in the future.

A change of location from my place of birth Mönchengladbach to Düsseldorf in 2000 led me to part-time a 2-year Shiatsu training followed by a 2-year Shiatsu training at the YoShi Shiatsu School in Düsseldorf.

I had gotten to know Shiatsu at a weekend seminar and immediately felt that I wanted to learn more about it. For me it was something like love at first sight. That's how I got to know the YoShi Shiat School in Düsseldorf.

Also at the YoShi-Shiatsuschule, Düsseldorf, I completed a 3-year yoga teacher training part-time. During this 7-year training period, I was able to further develop my personality profile. I gained new insights through constant training. I had found my calling .

After a few years of working as an office clerk, I felt that I didn't want to sit at my desk and work on paper until I retired. Rather, I was interested in personal contact with people - putting myself in their place and accompanying them on their life path. I developed the ability to empathize.

In addition, I have always enjoyed working independently and creatively. Initiative and a large amount of freedom are important values for me.

There is a new beginning in every crisis. So I was at a crossroads! After 19 professional years in the public sector fell my post restructuring victim and I was constantly placed where just up was needed. That wasn't exactly motivating. As was for me the time has come to break new ground. At this point in time I was 44 years old and I was starting a new phase of life in which I could realize myself. I gave up my permanent position and entered completely new territory. I fulfilled my heart's desire.

So I was pushed in the direction that is my calling. I dared to go NEW PATHS and founded my INSTITUT DELPHIN.

https://www.institut-delphin.de/

Dolphins have always fascinated me. They are available for healing and even used in Florida for the treatment of sick children.

They stand for polarity: day and night, good and bad, relaxation and tension, yin and yang (the principles of Chinese medicine). So everyone unites two sides in himself and has to find his own rhythm in the change of opposites.

Yoga and Shiatsu have expanded my consciousness.

Now I am living my dream, which I had already started part-time.

In search

Often the first vocational training is not necessarily what your own task in life is. Often the children are led by their parents in a certain professional direction because their own imagination is still missing at a young age. Later it can turn out that the profession you have learned is not really fulfilling. During the day you only have to do your duty and in the evening you deal with topics and activities that are fun.

At first I only attended courses in spinal gymnastics, which made my body more flexible. Then, with autogenic training, I got to know my body more deeply and consciously.

I discovered **yoga very** quickly , a way in which many aspects are united.

Relaxation and inner balance

There are different methods to find relaxation and inner balance.

In this book I write in the female form, although male readers are of course also addressed. First, I would like to go into *yoga* .

Yoga should be learned in a course under professional guidance. Anyone who seriously wants to make positive changes should also take part in yoga courses in the long term so that individual professional support is guaranteed.

It is important to convey to the participants that it is the goal of yoga to develop a sense of one's own body   and his own n perceive   limits. Therefore everyone should feel for themselves how long they want to and can stay in the individual exercises (asanas). It makes little sense to set a certain duration - as is practiced by some yoga teachers. So I have a lot of long-term participants who trust in my support.

In addition to attending the course, I recommend regular practice at home. It is important that I find a place in my apartment where I can be undisturbed for the duration of my yoga session (ideally 60 minutes). On the phone should e.g. B. the answering machine be switched on. It should be a place that I have set up comfortably and appropriately and that I like to retreat to. A yoga mat with a yoga pillow is recommended. Maybe I can light a candle and change the room air with an essential oil in a fragrance lamp. Scents have very individual effects on mind and soul - thus also on the chakras.

Yoga works on …

● **Physical level**

Hatha Yoga is widespread here in the West. In the exercises of Hatha Yoga, that is: physical exercises (asanas), breathing exercises (pranajama) and concentration (meditation), the deep muscles are gently strengthened. Through regular practice, the entire body becomes firmer - h auptsächlich by expansion, but also by strength exercises. The "yoga beginner" experiences her limits in terms of flexibility and breath control.

Every yoga student has very individual strengths and weaknesses. As a good yoga teacher, this must be balanced out and accompanied individually. Many beginners have problems adjusting their breathing during the exercises. But that is what makes the difference to other forms of movement. Yoga is a combination of movement, breathing and concentration.

With a little practice an expanded body awareness and a deep calm of the flow of thoughts develop. If a participant's thoughts cannot calm down, I can tell because she is not doing the exercise correctly. A good example of this is when she cannot stand quietly on one leg - as can be the case with the "tree".

By learning the breathing exercises (e.g. alternating breathing), the participant becomes more relaxed. The release of stress hormones decreases, the pulse calms down and breathing becomes calmer, the muscles relax.

Concentrating on the breath - especially the long and deep exhalation - creates a deep inner calm. Ideally, the thoughts come to rest. This can also help you to keep your inner balance in stressful situations in everyday life or to find it again quickly. **The aim of yoga is to lead a life in the here and now.** This means to be completely with the thoughts of what I am doing at the moment. Not to think about the past, because I can't change it anymore. But also not to the future, but to be completely absorbed in the respective activity - also known as "flow".

Yoga also encourages the right and left hemispheres to work together. D.Through the power of thoughts, I can alleviate mental disorders. If, for example, I feel pain or tension in my shoulders or neck, I can - if I have learned it through mindfulness training - direct my thoughts and my breathing there and thus alleviate the symptoms.

But the power of thought can do much more. The way we think is how we create our reality. Anyone who consciously decides to focus their attention on something positive actually experiences more and more pleasant things. Then problems suddenly turn into opportunities. Another effect can be that we suddenly have more energy and confidence to cope with a difficult situation.

This is the ancient spiritual law of attraction. Then success, happiness and a large social network move into our lives. We can be grateful for that. We feel less stress. Tension and pain can be relieved. Gratitude and positive thinking are the keys to a more fulfilling life.

● **Mental level**

The search for the meaning of life is an elementary question that probably everyone asks.

Where is my place in my life? What fills me What fills my life Where do I find quality of life for myself?

The way of life is decisive.

Would I like to lead a life in a partnership and start a family or would I rather stay single and enjoy my freedoms.

Is my career crucial for me? Then I should do what I like to do. This is how I prevent psychosomatic illnesses.

Physical symptoms are often related to emotional problems such as stress, overwork (or underwork) and fear. Because soul and body influence each other.

Physical illness can result from dissatisfaction. If I feel good, physical complaints will also go away. That is the approach of yoga. Well-being and inner balance are promoted by yoga and the self-healing powers are stimulated.

In summary it can be said: **Yoga is a spiritually spiritual** path of **experience to the self** and goes hand in hand with a personality development.

The closer we get to our inner selves, the more happiness we feel in our lives. Our wish in life is to be happy.

" Two things give the soul the greatest strength: trust in the truth and trust in oneself " Seneca (approx. 4 BC - 65 AD), Roman philosopher

Yoga from an Eastern perspective

As mentioned at the beginning of the previous chapter, I described yoga from the western perspective.

In the Eastern tradition the spiritual aspect is very pronounced. So that we understand each other correctly, yoga is **not a** religion, but a philosophy, a way of life. It's about finding inner peace within yourself. By training in mindfulness, everyday life becomes more conscious.

Regardless of any religion, there is always a belief in a higher power - no matter what its name is. Nothing happens "just like that" in life. Everything has a purpose. Even if the meaning of an event can often only be seen in retrospect.

Kundalini yoga and chakras

The type of yoga that deals with the chakras is called Kundalini Yoga and is very spiritual.

In the following I would like to give a brief, technical introduction to this:

Kundalini is the serpentine power, which according to ancient knowledge - as it is handed down through Hinduism - rests at the end of the spine and can rise through the central *channel* in the *Sushumna* when it is awakened. Nachfolgend you caneven deeper intothis boarding topic.

In the spine are fine-material (astral) channels (Nadi) - ver-parable with the nervous system in the spinal column. These channels have a wide variety of functions. So there are two nadis that are active when breathing. The air flows in and out through them. These nadis are called *Ida* and *Pingala*. Between these two nadis lies the *sushumna*. It is the central channel in the subtle body (*astral body*). The chakras are in the sushumna. It is the only nadi that connects all six chakras with the crown chakra. The subject of the chakras is very extensive. Read more about this in the following chapters.

In the sushumna there is another very fine nadi: *chitrini.* It is *the* actual tube in which Kundalini rises.

This process is only possible for yoga students with the help of various cleansing exercises, postures, breathing exercises and mudras (special hand positions).

The healing power of the mudras

In the following I would like to briefly discuss mudras. The whole subject is very extensive and based on scientific knowledge. It would go beyond the scope of this book. I therefore declare only a very common Mudra as in meditation out leads is.

The tips of the thumb and forefinger are touching. This finger position is known as the *Gyan Mudra.* It can be practiced from a minute to a maximum of half an hour. It is important that it is carried out with dedication. The elements air and fire are united. It's a very meaningful gesture. Great masters like Gautama Buddha, Jesus Christ, Bhagwan Krishna and other divine souls have already practiced them with great regularity.

These simple practice of Gyan Mudra brings the practitioner has a great benefit. This is so diverse and impressive that I quote below from the book "The Healing Power of Mudras": "If it is practiced for a long time, it gradually strengthens all tendons and blood vessels without medication or external aids. Mental strength increases and memory also gradually improves. Persistent practice of this mudra can cure sleep disorders and insomnia over time. When practiced over a long period, it exerts imperceptibly an extraordinary healing effect on the tiny Sin n esnervenzellen from the human's brain-.Significant changes have been observed in people's thinking. Regular practice of the Gyan Mudra can cure a variety of mental illnesses. "

In summary it can be said that the Gyan Mudra improves memory and the ability to concentrate enormously. It relieves irritability and leads to inner calm.

The position of the fingers when breathing alternately

In preparation for alternating breathing, the left hand rests on the left knee in the Gyan Mudra. In the right hand, the index finger and middle finger are bent. The thumb lightly touches the right nostril and the ring finger lightly touches the left nostril.

Alternate breathing then begins by releasing the left nostril and exhaling the old air completely on the left first. Then inhale again on the left and close the left nostril with the ring finger. The right nostril is released and thereby exhaled. Then inhale on the right and exhale on the left. This corresponds to 1 round. Alternating breathing is over after 12 rounds, with breathing out twice as long as breathing in.

I n my yoga hours I will from my participants often wondered how the correct finger position in the exchange-breathing is and whether it does not matter whether which fingers are used.

There are physical and energetic reasons for holding the fingers in alternating breathing:

Physically : It is the most relaxed finger position. Muscle tension would be required to stretch the fingers. When the fingers are bent, they are completely relaxed.

Energetic : Every finger has an energetic meaning:

● The little finger stands for **Rajas** (passion and dynamism).

● The ring finger stands for *sattwa* (purity and balance).

● The middle finger stands for *tamas* (darkness and indolence).

● The index finger stands for *ego* (I- relatedness).

● The thumb stands for **Brahman** (The Goddess).

The two purest finger (ring finger and thumb) are b enutzt. The energy of the right thumb corresponds to the energy of Pingala Nadi (right nostril, warming breath), the energy of the right ring finger that of Ida Nadi (left nostril, cooling breath). The ego finger is kept bent because the ego is supposed to bow. Likewise, the middle finger is bent. Both fingers should not point to the Ajna (forehead) chakra, as they could drain its energy. Nevertheless , some yoga schools teach to put the index finger on the Ajna Chakra because it can make concentration easier for beginners.

Chakras - the seven centers of power

The chakra teaching comes from the Indian yoga tradition, which is thousands of years old. The Sanskrit word " *chakra* " means something like wheel. It can be translated as "energy vortex" or "center of power". From a neurophysiological point of view, the chakras are connected to a network of fine channels like a kind of nerve plexus. Chakras are the energy centers in the body. Each chakra is connected to certain organs, glands and tissues via the fine channels. It is said that the chakras absorb the universal life energy (in Indian "Prana"; in Chinese medicine "Qi") and distribute it in the body.

Certain yoga exercises (asanas) can activate the flow of energy in the chakras. A chakra is called activated when the principle associated with it is accepted as a learning task in everyday life and its quality can be lived.

In addition to special yoga exercises (asanas), we

used special chakra images (according to Harish Johari) in our yoga teacher training and meditated on them later. Colors, shapes and the respective sound of the chakra are supported. With this activity alone, I was able to gain a wide range of experiences with the respective chakras .

We have dealt extensively with each of the seven chakras. This allowed me to develop my personality and my life has changed fundamentally.

In the following I would like to share my experiences with you, dear readers, in order to explain the chakras to you in more detail.

1st chakra: root or base chakra (Muladhara chakra)

The 1st chakra, the **root or base chakra** (**Muladhara chakra** ; Mula = root, adhara = support) sits on the coccyx and lower part of the sacrum, on the pelvic floor.

Our life force is stored in this area. Spiritually it is referred to as Kundalini and symbolically represented in the form of a snake that is coiled up in a spiral at the end of the spine. You can through meditation, intensive repetition of mantras or yoga Ü be awakened exercises and ascend to the higher chakras.

It is the **first level of consciousness** , the physical being.

Through the root chakra we take in the magnetic earth energy. It is the **earth element** , the **odor s meaningful** assigned the bones and teeth, spine, and the entire colon to the rectum. It is also related to the structure of the blood.

When I meditate, I feel a warm feeling on my tailbone, as if something is rising up my spine. The aim of meditation on the Muladhara Chakra is to promote health and the release of tension in the body and mind .

As the name suggests, it has to do with basis / strength and also with basic trust. Stress-related illnesses, varicose veins and osteoporosis indicate a disorder. A person who has a strong 1st chakra has a great deal of basic trust in himself and in his abilities, has both feet on the ground and masters his everyday life with strength, joy and confidence. He has material security, money and work.

In aromatherapy, carnation, rose, jasmine, patchouli, sandalwood and cedar support the development.

In everyday life, physical activity, lots of fresh air, nature, gardening, foot massages, walking barefoot, calf and thigh irrigation and, last but not least, everything that is **red** (clothing / objects) supports the root chakra. Rhythmic music (drumming) is also helpful.

In yoga lessons all standing postures influence (because of grounding, earth energy, roots); everything that acts on the feet, knees, legs, pelvis, sacrum, coccyx area and all prevent the Muladhara chakra.

2nd chakra: sacral or sexual chakra Svadhistana chakra)

The 2nd chakra, the **sacral or sexual chakra (Svadhistana chakra** ; Svadhisthana = sweetness, loveliness) is located between the pubic bone and the navel. As with any chakra, there is a front and a corresponding back chakra.

Connected to it are the pelvic area, the sacrum, the genital and abdominal organs, the gonads, the immune system and the lumbar spine.

The sacral chakra regulates and harmonizes the fluid balance and the blood circulation in the body and ensures detoxification via the bladder and kidneys.

It is the **second level of consciousness** , the transmission of being. There is the abode of the self; it is the meeting of I and you - both in me too - so ultimately the meeting with myself; take and give. It is assigned to the **water element** and the **sense of taste** and also stands for sensuality, sexuality and reproduction.

I often meet people who have lower back complaints (sacrum and sacroiliac joint = SI joint). These complaints can be alleviated well with certain yoga exercises or with a Shiatsu treatment - which I will go into in more detail later. Frequent bladder infections can also be related to a blocked sacral chakra.

A strong Svadhisthana chakra shows itself in flowing movements, in harmony in relationships, in creativity, joie de vivre and vitality. The goal of meditation on the Svadhisthana chakra is to detach yourself from sensual pleasure and the ego. Ylang-ylang, sandalwood, bergamot and bitter orange support the development in aromatherapy.

In everyday life, everything that has to do with water supports you: a walk by the lake, bathing, swimming, steam bath, a lot of drinking. Creativity is encouraged through the visual arts and dancing; the sensuality awakened by fragrant body oils and aromatic baths.

Everything that is **orange** (clothes / objects) has a positive effect on the Svadhisthana chakra.

29

In yoga classes, all standing postures influence all bending forward; everything that affects the pelvic area, sacrum, hip joints and lumbar spine, the Svadhisthana chakra.

3rd chakra: umbilical chakra or solar plexus
(manipura chakra)

The 3rd chakra, the **umbilical chakra or solar plexus (Manipura chakra** ; Manipura = shining jewel) is located on the upper abdomen and accordingly on the back of the body.

The vegetative nervous system and digestive organs such as stomach / spleen, liver / gall bladder, small intestine and pancreas are connected to it.

It is assigned the personality, the ego, power, self-confidence and feelings like longing, compassion and sensitivity. When two strong personalities meet, it can lead to arguments and "power struggles".

It creates the connection between thinking and feeling and is the chakra of the middle of the body.

It is the **third level of consciousness**, the order of

being. It is assigned to the **fire element** and **seeing.**

Disorders can manifest themselves in tantrums, heartburn, pain in the upper abdomen, a lack of assertiveness and inner overstimulation.

A strong 3rd chakra shows itself in good nervous condition, good sleep and awareness of one's own strength.

When I meditated, I sometimes felt like I had a lump in my stomach. The aim of meditation on the Manipura chakra is to overcome physical desire. Inspired teaching is to be mentioned as a special power.

In aromatherapy, lavender, lemon, bergamot, rosemary and anise have a supportive effect on development.

In everyday life, deep abdominal breathing, short sunbathing, fire (fireplace, campfire, candles) and soulful music provide support.

Everything that is **yellow** (clothing / objects) has a positive effect on the Manipura chakra.

In yoga classes, all twisting exercises and everything that affects the abdominal organs affect the manipura chakra.

4th Chakra:
Heart Chakra (Anahata Chakra)

The 4th chakra, the **heart chakra (anahata chakra** ; anahata = not chipped, undamaged) has its place above the sternum to the cervical fossa and accordingly on the back of the body.

Connected to it are the heart, lungs , bronchi, blood circulation, skin, arms and hands, upper back, shoulders and the thymus gland (immune system).

It stands for openness, spontaneity, warmth of the heart, affection, love, security and healing. That is why a Shiatsu treatment has a lot to do with the heart chakra. It is a special ability to let the love energy flow from the middle of the hand and thus to stimulate the self-healing powers.

It establishes the connection between the lower three chakras (material world / body) and the upper three chakras (mental, spiritual world / spirit).

It is the **fourth level of consciousness** , the Emotional Self.

It is assigned to the **air element** and the **buttons** .

Blockages in the heart chakra can be contact difficulties, loneliness, breathing difficulties, frequent colds, fears, emotional stress and cardiac arrhythmias.

A strong anahata chakra shows itself in inner harmony, in overcoming selfish thinking and acting, in comprehensive unconditional love, in the willingness to love yourself and others. It is easy to take responsibility for others and to lovingly accept yourself despite weaknesses and mistakes. From the heart chakra, when stimulated by the Kundalini, we are able to know what others are feeling by experiencing these feelings within ourselves. This is how I perceive physical tension in my yoga course participants by feeling them in myself. During Shiatsu treatment, it is therefore very important that I delimit myself energetically so that I do not take on the client's disorders.

While meditating, I feel a warm feeling in the middle of my chest, but at times also a sharp pain.

Aromatherapy uses rose, mint and sage to support development.

In everyday life, the Anahata chakra is strengthened when we pamper ourselves and give gifts, go outdoors a lot and let the green of meadows and forests affect us; when we care for others, are open to the problems of others and show compassion to other living beings (including animals).

Touching and hugging other people, Shiatsu and everything that is **green** (clothing / objects / lots of green plants in the home) also has a positive effect on the anahata chakra.

In yoga classes, all backbends, rotations, exercises for shoulders, thoracic spine, arms and hands and everything that affects the cardiovascular system (e.g. sun salutation) affect the Anahata chakra.

5th chakra: throat or larynx chakra (Vishudda chakra)

The 5th chakra, the **throat or larynx chakra (Vishudda chakra;** Vishuddhi = cleanse) extends from the upper breastbone over the entire neck. Its center is in the throat and accordingly on the back of the body.

The neck, larynx, jaw, esophagus and windpipe, breathing, voice, neck and shoulders, ears and thyroid (metabolism, nervous system) are connected to it.

Communication, word awareness (being able to express oneself, understanding and being understood), inspiration, mental strength, expression of creativity and musicality are assigned to it. It is important for communication, the way we express ourselves, for inspiration and for mental strength.

The throat chakra is connected to the sexual

chakra, which is why one can feel an orgasm in the throat.

It is the **fifth level of consciousness**, the expression of being.

It is assigned to the **etheric element** (Akasha) and **hearing** .

Disorders are: Difficulty expressing feelings and thoughts in words; Inhibitions, shyness, no access to the inner voice, sore throat and tonsillitis; Sensation of lump and tightness in the throat; Speech disorders, e.g. B. Stuttering; Inflammation of the oral cavity, gums and jaw; Pain in the cervical spine, neck and shoulders; Over- / underactive thyroid and associated disorders such as B. Nervousness / lack of drive; the feeling of not belonging.

A strong Vishuddha chakra shows itself in expression, fluency, communication skills and a beautiful voice. The conscious use of words showed in me that I was direct, but kindly say what

I think.

The expression of being and uniqueness should be mentioned as a special force.

The aim of meditation on the Vishuddha chakra is knowledge from the past.

Eucalyptus, camphor, sage and peppermint support the development of aromatherapy.

In everyday life, the Vishuddha chakra is strengthened by learning foreign languages, attending rhetoric courses, writing a diary, vacationing at the sea or a (blue) lake, vocal exercises with vowels and mantras, music lessons and singing lessons, singing along in the choir, expressing one's opinion.

Everything that is **light blue** (clothing / objects) has a positive effect on the Vishuddha chakra. In yoga classes, all backbends and inversions, all exercises for the cervical spine and neck, and the lion posture affect the Vishuddha chakra.

6th chakra: Third eye or forehead chakra (Ajna chakra)

The 6th chakra, the **third eye or forehead chakra (Ajna chakra** ; Ajna = perceive) is located in the middle between the eyebrows or on the upper neck, where the skull and spine are connected.

Connected to it are the sensory organs eyes, ears and nose, the sinuses, the brain, the pituitary gland (pituitary gland) and thus the entire hormonal and nervous system.

Intuition, wisdom, knowledge, perception, fantasy, imagination and self-knowledge are assigned to him.

It is the **sixth** level of consciousness, the knowledge of being.

It is associated with the **Supreme Element** and **Intuition.**

Disturbances are noticeable in: concentration and learning difficulties, lack of insight, restless mind, fears and delusions, mental confusion, headaches and migraines, brain diseases, eye and ear problems, chronic. Colds and sinus infections, nervous system diseases and neurological disorders.

A strong forehead chakra shows itself in good memory and the ability to concentrate, good intuition and knowledge of higher realities beyond everyday consciousness, supernatural perception (telepathy), good imagination, mental clarity and self-knowledge.

Telepathy should be mentioned as a special power. During the meditation on the 3rd eye, I felt a connection to a loved one who was in a difficult situation at that time.

Another example is that I am thinking of a loved one and then he calls. There is a spiritual connection. Everything that happens can also be influenced by our thoughts. It is the law of cause and effect or the power of our subconscious.

Yoga makes life easier because solutions to everyday problems can be found more easily. Solution-oriented thinking sets in.

When I meditate, I feel a tickling sensation in the middle of the forehead. The aim of meditation on the Ajna chakra is unity and spiritual guidance.

In aromatherapy, lavender, jasmine, mint, rosemary and lemongrass support development.

In everyday life the Ajna chakra is strengthened by studying philosophical and religious writings, dealing with one's dreams and meditation.

Everything that is **indigo blue** (clothing / objects) has a positive effect on the Ajna chakra.

In yoga classes, all inverse postures, eye exercises,

visualization exercises, alternating breathing and kapalabhati (rapid abdominal breathing) influence the Ajna chakra.

7th Chakra:
Crown or Crown Chakra
(Sahasrara Chakra)

The 7th chakra, the **crown or crown chakra (Sahasrara chakra** ; Sahasrara = thousandfold, thousandfold), is represented as a thousand-petalled lotus. It sits on the apex of the head, its center being the posterior fontanel.

Connected to it are the midbrain and the pineal gland (epiphysis), which ensures the sleep-wake rhythm.

Spirituality, knowledge of God, trust in God, religiosity, perfection and enlightenment are assigned to him.

No individual organs are assigned to it, but it has a protective effect on the entire organism.

When I meditate, I sometimes feel a vibration under the top of my skull. The aim of meditation on the Sahasrara chakra is the liberation of the mind, pure being, the higher self, living in the here and now. It is **beyond consciousness** , **pure being** and basically not a chakra, but the point at which the body is overcome.

Disturbances of the crown chakra show up in: attachment to the material world; a feeling of lack, emptiness, and dissatisfaction; World Pain; Dullness; mental exhaustion; Negation of creativity; Immunodeficiency; Nerve ailments; Signs of paralysis; Cancer diseases; Difficulty falling asleep and staying asleep; lack of connection between body and mind.

When the Sahasrara chakra is free from interference, deep inner peace can be felt, spiritual understanding and self-realization are present. Provided that all other chakras are also fully developed and free from interference, enlightenment and perfection will occur.

The unity with the absolute is to be mentioned as a special force.

Incense, mint and clove support the development

of aromatherapy.

In everyday life, the Sahasrara chakra is strengthened by climbing mountain peaks and sweeping views.

White or **purple** clothes, objects or flowers have a positive effect on the Sahasrara chakra.

In yoga lessons, all inversion postures, but above all quiet exercises, meditations, the mantra OM and exercises to perceive the aura strengthen the Sahasrara chakra.

Only the great masters like Jesus or Buddha are enlightened. In addition to the experiences already described, I have come so far that I have become calmer inside and have a constant feeling of happiness and love in me. The spirituality in me has grown and I want to continue into light and love. I want to keep love inside me all the time

I would like to close the chapter on the chakras with a small, philosophical verse from Ursula Polaczek, with whom I began my training in the group:

The light has awakened in the heart

And now shines all the time day and night.

The rays draw large circles

And bring people on a journey.

You hike a lot and have time -

But then get ready

to go to the land of love.

The meaning of the mantras

With the 1st chakra I spoke of intensive repetition of a mantra in connection with Kundalini awakening. Therefore, I would now like to briefly go into the meaning of the mantras.

Mantras (Man = think, ponder, linger; Tra = cross over, free, save) are mostly sung in Sanskrit (the oldest language in the world and used in India for thousands of years for spiritual purposes). This may sound strange to our ears and takes getting used to, but it has a very special power. They help to balance physical imbalances, relax the mind, calm the emotions and open the heart.

It's worth getting involved in chanting a mantra even if we don't understand the words. It depends on the vibrations and the associated energy that a mantra has. These have a direct effect on the nervous system. Chanting (chanting) mantras is a very beautiful, peaceful method of expanding consciousness. It conveys joie de vivre and helps you to come to terms with yourself and just to BE - to forget everything around you. It helps to open the heart and awaken inner feelings of love, humility, and adoration.

The best known mantra is OM - the most original of all mantras. OM actually consists of the letters AU   M.
AUM represents all trinities: creation - preservation - destruction, past - present - future.

In my training we dealt extensively with the Gayatri mantra. It is the most sacred prayer in India - an invocation to the divine light. When chanting, a strongly noticeable energy unfolds.

The Gayatri mantra

" Oṃ bhūr bhuvaḥ svaḥ
tát savitúr váreniyaṃ
bhárgo devásya dhīmahi <
dhíyo yó naḥ pracodáyāt"

Translation and meaning of the Gayatri mantra

Om - We meditate on the shine and radiance of the adorable highest divine reality, the source of all being, the physical, astral and causal plane. May the Supreme Divine Being illuminate our minds and awaken our discernment so that we may experience the absolute truth.

The power of colors

When describing the seven chakras, I wrote which colors activate each chakra. Now I would like to go into more detail about the power of colors from the perspective of TCM (Traditional Chinese Medicine).

Colors subconsciously affect us by changing our mood. Each color affects our body differently because it has different vibrations.

Blue
calms you down

It is the purest and deepest color. According to the doctrine of chakras, BLUE corresponds to the 6th chakra and is assigned to the **water element** in TCM .

Blue puts our nerves into sleep mode, loosens muscles and inhibits inflammation. It looks cool, clears the mind and promotes prudent action.

green

harmonized

We combine green with nature and spring. In TCM, GREEN is assigned to the **wood element** . It relaxes the **eyes** and calms the soul; invigorates and refreshes. Mood swings can be balanced out. It has a detoxifying effect on the body, loosens the muscles in the chest and strengthens the heart and lungs. According to the chakra doctrine, it is assigned to the heart chakra.

yellow

is optimistic

Yellow makes you happy immediately. In TCM, YELLOW is assigned to the **earth element** . It has a stimulating effect on the nerves and the **digestive organs** . Accordingly, according to the chakra doctrine, it is assigned to the solar plexus.

orange

activated

The sunny tone gives strength and joie de vivre (as can also be found in the 2nd chakra). There is no equivalent in TCM. Orange stimulates the appetite and is therefore suitable for dishes.

purple

inspired

Purple strengthens the determination and helps to achieve mental balance. In the chakra doctrine we connect LILA with the 7th chakra. There is no equivalent in TCM.

red

gives power

The intense color gives us energy and vitality. RED stimulates blood pressure and circulation - so red socks can provide a remedy for cold feet. A red sweater can give us energy for the day if we are still feeling tired in the morning. In the chakra doctrine, RED is assigned to the root chakra and in TCM to the fire element.

The color assignment to the chakras can be different depending on the textbook. I assigned the colors as I learned in my training.

Qi Gong - source of energy

As I mentioned at the beginning of my book, there are different methods of finding relaxation and inner balance.

Therefore, I would now like to go into **Qi Gong** .

Qi Gong is a simple and at the same time intensive way to bring body, mind and soul into harmony. Qi Gong has a tradition of over 2000 years in Asia.

There are numerous scientific studies on Qi Gong. They came to the conclusion that regular and persistent Qi Gong practice strengthens the immune system and regulates the circulatory system. The nervous system, especially the vegetative one, is stabilized. A strengthening of the function of the breathing system and harmonization of the emotional part of the psyche have also been proven.

Qi Gong is a complex system of exercises that emerged from the tradition of Taoism, Buddhism and Chinese medicine. It means "cultivating the Qi". Qi is the life energy that, according to the traditional Chinese view, exists throughout the cosmos and also in the human body.

Qi Gong stimulates the self-healing powers, gives the body flexibility and suppleness, stimulates the flow of energy and leads to the gradual dissolution of physical and mental tensions.

If the Qi flows harmoniously, we feel healthy and balanced, we feel a strong vitality and inner strength. In addition, the perception of ourselves and of our daily environment changes. We become more sensitive to our own bodies, perceive the moods of our fellow human beings more quickly and become more receptive to events in our surroundings.

Qi Gong is usually practiced while standing. The body is stabilized through prolonged standing in connection with slow, deep breathing. In the imagination, the feet are firmly rooted in the ground. This can create the feeling of penetrating deeper and deeper into the earth. The breath becomes calmer and finer. Its power fills the whole lower abdomen. The deep breath massages and cleanses the internal organs. A feeling of warmth spreads in the center and, after some practice, fills the entire body.

Those who get involved in attending a Qi Gong course can notice different reactions, especially as a beginner. At first, the very slow movement may seem strange. Most people are used to the fact that everything always has to happen quickly. Many are inwardly driven, they unconsciously sense the strong contrasts and would like to run away. The tension can build up in someone's body to the point that symptoms such as initial pain in the muscles and even coughing fits - the tension is released. Other signs may include internal tremors or an impulse to cry. From the point of view of psychology, these are positive reactions of the body. It is always worthwhile to continue with the practice, as there is a developmental process taking place in every Qi Gong practitioner.

The deeper the practitioner penetrates into the practice of Qi Gong, the more they perceive that a fine energetic field also exists around the body. Everyone's energy field (the aura) extends as far as the outstretched arms of each practitioner. When many practitioners stand in a circle, a closed energy circle is created and the energy flows very well overall. Harmony and warmth as well as deep inner peace can be felt. If possible, it should be avoided that individual practitioners leave the circle during the exercise cycle. This would create an energetic hole and weaken the overall effect of Qi Gong.

The effect of Qi Gong can be felt over the long term. Inner peace and balance can continue the next day and maybe even longer. This is how Qi Gong works in our everyday life and we can better perform our everyday tasks.

Shiatsu - relaxation massage

Another method to find relaxation and inner balance is a Shiatsu relaxation massage.

In contrast to the relaxation techniques yoga and Qi Gong already mentioned, it is a passive but very beneficial variant.

You lie in comfortable clothes on a soft mat on the floor and just let it happen. I am then the active one.

In the following I would like to explain to you, dear readers, what you can expect from a Shiatsu relaxation massage.

Before I start a relaxation massage, I have a detailed conversation - at an initial appointment - to get an idea of the physical or psychological impairments. That makes it easier for me to get started with the subsequent Shiatsu treatment. As a supplementary remedy, I use the so-called "Hara diagnosis". I feel different areas on your stomach that are assigned to the organs. Depending on whether they feel soft or hard, I will then know how to design my Shiatsu relaxation massage.

The organs are in turn assigned to the meridians (energy channels). By working with finger, thumb and ball of the hand pressure techniques on the corresponding meridian, your energy is harmonized. I tend to work on the meridians where the tsubos (energy points) can be easily indented, i.e. where there is too little energy, than on muscle hardening.

Shiatsu is based on the theory that the energy flows from where there is too much energy (i.e. there is hardening or blockages) to where there is too little energy. This can relieve muscle tension.

During a Shiatsu relaxation massage, I work your whole body: your stomach, arms and legs, head and back. I also use gentle stretches and joint rotations. A Shiatsu relaxation massage consists of calm and flowing movements.

It is a relaxing and stress-relieving body work that stimulates your self-healing powers. You can enjoy the Shiatsu relaxation massage for 60 minutes.

I have received very good feedback from clients with migraines or back pain.

Shiatsu is not a healing treatment, but a help for self-help in order to support one's own strength for self-healing.

Shiatsu is based on the basic ideas of traditional Chinese medicine.

Meridians

In the previous chapter I wrote about meridians. I would now like to describe this in more detail.

You already know that meridians are energy channels. Like the visible channels - veins, arteries, lymph and nerve tracts - these run through the whole body and lie flat under the skin in the subcutaneous tissue.

The meridians are connected to the organs. By feeling a lack of energy or a blockage in Shiatsu with my hands, I can act on it in a targeted manner. This has a preventive effect on the corresponding organ.

For example, when a cold is approaching, I can detect a lack of energy in the lung meridian and treat it accordingly through Shiatsu. This can have the effect that the cold either does not break out in the first place or with very strong symptoms, but the duration is shortened. Before a disease breaks out on an organic level, there is an imbalance in the energy distribution in the meridians. There is either too much or too little energy there.

Basic ideas of TCM

According to Traditional Chinese Medicine (TCM), body, soul and spirit are connected and form a unit.

A disturbance in one of the areas affects the others as well.

A balanced flow of energy in the body is important for health. If the flow of energy is disturbed or blocked, illness develops.

When the energy can flow freely, you are in balance and feel healthy.

As already mentioned, life energy (Qi) flows in the meridians. Qi is the essence of life.

"' Man lives in the midst of qi, and the qi fills

man. Everything needs Qi in order to live, 'says a

Chinese text from the 4th century. "

(Quote from: "Atlas of Holistic Healing")

The five element doctrine

According to Chinese scriptures, the meridian system is based on the historically older five-element theory.

When describing the colors, I already mentioned the five-element theory according to TCM. Therefore I would like to continue the description here.

Also in the description of the chakras I mentioned the assignment to the elements. However, this is based on the Indian / Ayurvedic view - different from TCM.

But now to the TCM. Traditional Chinese Medicine knows the five elements that are associated with the seasons:

- **Wood** - spring

- **Fire** - summer

- **Earth** - late summer
- **Metal** - autumn and

- **Water** - winter

Corresponding meridians and thus also organs are assigned to the elements:

- **Wood -** gall bladder and liver M Eridian

- **Fire** - (there are two pairs of meridians):

- Cardiovascular system and triple heater as well
- Heart and small intestine meridian

- **Earth** - stomach and spleen meridians

- **Metal** - lung and D ickdarm meridian

- **Water** - bladder and kidney meridian

In Shiatsu I assume that there is an imbalance in the meridian that belongs to the season. That's why I always treat him with. Let's stick with our example from earlier. In autumn, the lung and colon meridian are always part of my Shiatsu relaxation massage. This is almost self-explanatory, because colds occur more frequently in autumn.

In addition, certain flavors are assigned to the elements:

● **Wood** - sour

● **Fire** - bitter

● **Earth** - cute

● **Metal** - sharp

● **Water** - salty

I make use of this assignment in the survey before the first Shiatsu relaxation massage .

When I know which flavor you prefer, I already have a clue for my treatment. Suppose you have a tendency to sweet foods, then I know that S he most likely a lack of energy in the earth element have.

These same S he intuitively by sweet foods. So in the Shiatsu relaxation massage I will treat the stomach and spleen meridians.

The sense organs are also assigned to the five elements according to traditional Chinese medicine :

● **Wood** -eyes

● **Fire** - tongue

● **Earth** - mouth

- **Metal**-nose

- **Water** -ear

By observing my client, I can see in which element there is a disorder.

For example, if you talk a lot and very quickly, you very likely have too much energy in the fire element.

Watery eyes can indicate a disturbance in the wood element, a runny nose (cold) can indicate a disturbance in the metal element and noises in the ears (tinnitus) can indicate a disturbance in the water element.

In addition to the sense organs, the body layers are also assigned to the elements:

- **Wood**- tendons

- **Fire** -vessels

- **Earth** - muscles, connective tissue

- **Metal** -skin

- **Water** - bones

Here I would like to name the varicose veins as an example, which indicate a weakness in the connective tissue and thus a weakness in the earth element.

I can also infer an energetic disturbance in the corresponding element from the emotions that predominate in a person:

- **Wood** - trouble

- **Fire** - joy

- **Earth** - worry / brooding

- **Metal** - grief

- **Water** - fear

Finally, I would like to talk about the sounds that are assigned to the elements:

- **Wood** - calling

- **Fire** - laughter

- **Earth** - singing

- **Metal** - wines n

- **Water** - sigh

For example, if I have someone in front of me who laughs very often - sometimes in situations where laughter is inappropriate - there is a high probability that they have too much energy in the fire element and, as a result, too little energy in the water element. So with a Shiatsu relaxation massage I would treat the water element with the bladder and kidney meridians.

There are many other equivalents to the five elements, but that is beyond the scope of this book.

TCM nutrition

From the point of view of TCM, all foods can function as medicaments. With proper nutrition we can not only achieve a harmonious relationship between yin and yang in the body and thus maintain a high level of vitality for life, but also prevent and heal diseases or support healing.

What is the difference between Chinese and Western dietetics?

The **Western** Nutrition emphasizes the nutrients from food, so the proportion of proteins, fats, carbohydrates, etc. It is particularly important, the content of vitamins, minerals and trace elements. Therefore, vital substance supplements have become more and more popular in recent years. The idea is always that the food should meet the body's need for nutrients.

I n the **Chinese** nutrition, attention is more on the prevention and cure of K laid rank units. In this way, an energetic imbalance - such as chronic fatigue, exhaustion or susceptibility to infection - can be recognized early before it can manifest itself as an illness.

Food and medicinal herbs are considered medicinal products. Knowledge of their health effects and energetic properties are therefore very important.

Many foods can build up energy directly, while others strengthen the inner core, heat the body or have a cooling effect. There are also foods that stir up diseases, such as B. Seafood or lamb, or create an "internal moisture" - this includes dairy products, sweets or cold food. Excessive consumption of these foods often leads to obesity or listlessness. Knowledge of the energetic and health effects of food and medicinal herbs is used in TCM as the basis for preventing or treating diseases effectively.

The digestive system and the interaction of the organs is very much appreciated. In other words, the structure of the inner center is a key point in TCM. When the digestive system is weakened, it is difficult for the body to absorb energy, no matter how rich in nutrients the food is. For this reason, there is a S chwer-point of TCM on building our midst.

In order to achieve special health effects, foods are often cooked together with medicinal herbs; the Chinese call it "healing food".

What do you mean with that?

Chinese herbs have a special healing effect. For this reason, normal foods or dishes, such as concentrated soups, are often cooked together with one or more herbs. Dad hrough can K rank units before ge beug t or de r healing process can be supported. Life energy and vitality can be built up and a long and healthy life can be maintained . Methods such as Qi Gong, Tai Chi or acupressure also provide support .

It is also important to know that there is a difference between *"**healing food and medicinal herbs**"*. The first is a food with herbs as an addition. Under the second, only herbs are meant as medicine.

The medicine is prescribed in China, meanwhile also in Germany, by Chinese doctors and naturopaths against various diseases. But everyone can prepare healing food for themselves. This easy implementation, which is possible on a daily basis, makes it easy to achieve lasting therapeutic effects.

The vital substance supplement from Sisel International contains herbs from **traditional Chinese medicine.** This makes it possible for those of you who are neither familiar with western nor with Chinese nutritional science to prevent diseases, build up your life energy and vitality and maintain a long and healthy life.

Yoga and Diet

A conscious life, which includes all of the above, also includes paying attention to my diet. For example , I do not use additives in food, such as flavor enhancers, and go shopping consciously. I also watch out for potentially questionable ingredients in personal care products and household cleaning products. I turn the bottle upside down and look up the ingredients.

But now back to the subject of "nutrition": The state of the mind is influenced by the type of food we eat and the way we eat it.

We humans are the only living things that eat, even when we are not hungry. In general, we live to eat and do not eat to live. When we eat for the palate, we overeat and suffer from digestive disorders that upset our system.

The yogi believes in harmony and eats d eshalb only to maintain his life. He's not eating too much or too little. He regards his body as the refuge for his spirit and protects himself from being overly spoiled. A yogi fills half of his stomach with pure (sattvic) food, a quarter with pure water and a quarter remains empty. He eats so much that he is full, but not so much that he feels sluggish and heavy. This corresponds to the findings of modern nutritional science.

There are no particular dietary requirements for someone starting asanas (physical exercises). After a period of practice, you will automatically crave natural food in the right amount. You don't have to become a vegetarian, but as you advance to the higher levels, a vegetarian diet becomes necessary.

Cheap foods:

Fruit:

A fruit diet has a calming effect on the constitution and is very desirable for yogis. It is a natural diet. Fruits are great sources of energy. Bananas, grapes, sweet oranges, apples, pomegranates, mangoes and dates are easily digestible fruits. Lemons have scurvy preventive properties and act as a blood tonic. Fruit juice contains vitamin C. Mangoes and milk are a very healthy combination. You can only live on milk and mangoes. The juice of pomegranates is cooling and very nutritious. Bananas are nutritious and invigorating. Fruits promote concentration and facilitate mental concentration.

Nourishing and sweet

Suitable foods are: cereals, milk, fresh and clarified butter (the Indian ghee), brown sugar, honey, ginger and various vegetables (except fennel and pulses). Vegetables that ripen above the ground are preferable to those that ripen underground because they can store more solar energy. Exceptions are beetroot and carrots. Barley is a good food for a yogi because it has a cooling effect. Nourishing and sweet, mixed with melted butter and milk, this promotes the body fluids and is pleasant for yogis.

In relation to our living space, a lacto-vegetarian diet is recommended that takes into account the need for sweets.

If we practice the breathing techniques of yoga (pranayama) intensively, we should eat more milk and butter at the beginning, because these exercises cause some turmoil in the nervous system and stimulate very strongly. Milk and butter then help to cool down and calm the body again. After a while, your body will get used to exercising and you can return to a less high-calorie diet.

The favorable foods, ie fruits and Nourishing and Sü ß to be as **tired of wiping food** referred. They bring clarity, joy, life energy and satisfaction.

It is important with what awareness the food is prepared. Loving thoughts while cooking enliven the prepared food.

All food contains a small amount of salt so that it no longer needs to be seasoned with salt. Salt arouses passion. By not using salt, no disturbances are caused. Eliminating salt helps control the tongue and mind, willpower is developed.

Unfavorable food

Since practicing can be very energizing, it makes sense to avoid food and beverages that stimulate additional stimulation, such as hot spices, paprika, radish, onions, garlic and chillies as well as all luxury foods such as coffee, tea and alcohol. They are called **Rajas Foods** . They strengthen the passion and heat up the body and mind. They make people opinionated, aggressive and impatient. However, if rather slow, sluggish and indifferent, can this food smittel eat in small amounts. Activate en sluggish people and bring s them more determination, activity impulses and assertiveness.

Few things are considered really unhealthy: foods that contain too much acid, salt or pepper, and those that are no longer fresh or spoiled.

Here, too, it is important for the quality of the food what mood the cook is in: if he is irritated, full of tension or angry, this is carried over to the prepared food.

The third group of foods that describe the effects on consciousness are the **Tamasic foods** . They make the mind and body tired, sluggish, negative and dull. They put a strain on the digestive system and favor diseases.

Tamasic foods include: Meat, mushrooms, onions and leeks, hard cheese, long-life milk, foods with preservatives, frozen and canned products, warmed up foods, instant and ready-made products, genetically modified and synthetic foods, vinegar, refined sugar, industrial manufactured salt and peanut products. This group also includes alcohol and drugs.

If the cook is tired, sluggish, lazy, behaves lethargic and is full of negative thoughts, this is carried over to the prepared food. This also happens when the kitchen is dirty.

Balanced and moderate

When we deal with yoga, it becomes increasingly clear that we are striving for balance and harmony. We become aware of what we overemphasize in our life and what things we have given too little space. We experience in body, soul and spirit that it is good for us to be balanced in everything. We develop a feeling for the choice of food and put our yogic meal together according to our temperament and constitution.

Diet for yogis therefore means nothing more than a balanced diet that is good for us and is good for us. But balanced also means not eating too much or too little.

Why meat is not so healthy: Pros and cons of meat

Whether you eat vegetarian or not, is a personal matter which of your tradition and your influenced habits and education.

However, meat is heavier in the stomach than vegetables and requires much more energy for digestion. It shifts the acid-base balance of the body towards the acidic. Meat excites passion and makes the mind restless. Last but not least, ethical questions come into play, at least whether we really want to support the sometimes unworthy practices of "meat production". Therefore we should at least pay attention to controlled rearing, and we should eat meat in moderation and in gratitude to the being who makes his life available to us.

And let's not forget: humans cannot be healthier than the products they eat! Life can only be sustained by the living - not the dead.

Nutritional situation today

Today's diet contains too much sugar, too much fat and too much salt.

Many eat one-sidedly. There is a lack of a balanced diet.

70% of all doctor visits are caused by nutritional errors

60% of all people suffer from overweight and lack of energy

40% suffer from vitamin deficiency

52% of all people in the western world die of malnutrition

We starve to death on full plates!

Minerals and trace elements

According to the classic doctrine, a balanced diet with the four main food groups fruit, vegetables, grains and animal protein is completely sufficient to provide us with everything the organism needs. Here, our food is assigned a lot more ingredients than they still contain after forced growth on impoverished soils, after storage and processing.

The daily requirement was also set at a level that ignored the increased requirements due to stress and environmental pollution. Where alternative medicine points out the importance of nutrient additives, it is played down again by representatives of official conventional medicine. The common consequence is that our bodies go hungry in the midst of an affluent society. While the supply of vitamins is considered sufficient in many cases, the supply of the full spectrum of minerals and trace elements is increasingly inadequate and prevents us from experiencing optimal health. This insight is now widely recognized as one of the most important since the existence of nutritional science.

My holistic health concept

At the time when my new phase of life began, I got to know from my parents a very effective vital substance supplement with herbs from traditional Chinese medicine, which strengthened me from within. So I was able to cope with this difficult upheaval. Gradually, I got to know other products from this company and became more and more convinced, because I felt a strength in me that drove me to prepare for my new phase of life despite the still difficult final phase in the public service.

Then I wanted to learn more about the Unternehmensphilosop h know ie. The **family company Sisel International** was founded in 2006 with the mission to develop and manufacture the world's most effective and toxin-free personal care products and dietary supplements. Did you know that your home can be one of the greatest threats to you and your family - just from the products you use every day?

Over 30 years ago discovered Tom Mower, sen., That in many common household care products precarious and hazardous chemicals partially contained . He found that many of the harsh chemicals used in industrial cleaners are also found in common household items for personal care.

These chemicals pose health risks to you and your family if they come in contact with your skin.

So he began a scientific research that would make history. He founded a research laboratory for much more effective and healthier products. Thus arose the *Mower - Mission* , a global community of active members, the health and wellness recommend. **For everyone who loves a vital and healthy life!**

The range includes body care, face care, hair care and the household sector. The program is rounded off by nutritional supplements rich in vital substances. Everything is manufactured by Sisel in its own state-of-the-art production facility with 400,000 square meters based on current, scientific

studies. The products are free from animal experiments and genetically modified organisms, safe, effective and environmentally friendly, marked with the Sisel Safe® logo.
100% toxin free - 100% innovative - 100% effective

Sisel International is a global industry leader. Founders Tom Mower Sr. and Tom Mower Jr. have been leaders in the health and wellness industry for over 30 years.

The term SISEL is an abbreviation for the English terms:

Science, Innovation, Success, Energy and Longevity.

In German this stands for:

Science, innovation, success, energy and longevity.

These are the basic principles of the company.

The company's founder, scientist and biochemist Tom Mower Sr. had a vision: to create health, prosperity and happiness for everyone around the world. Everyone can help spread the Mower Mission.

https://sisel.net/delphin66

All of this fits wonderfully into my holistic health concept, in which I show you individual solutions to maintain your health, improve your fitness and optimize the aging process. These are exclusive topics for better health and a more vital life.

The 4 phases of nutrient research

1st phase: Linus Pauling phase

Vitamins as **monopreparations** in high
doses. One advantage is often
m bought it another disadvantage.

2nd phase: Combination preparations

Complexity and interdependence of
vital substances: calcium, for
example, has magnesium as an opponent.

**3rd phase: beginning of the 21st century:
secondary plant substances**

E inbindung of all vital substances in
P flanzenwirkstoffen. In the right

proportion, as nature provides us with.
We need over 70 different
vital substances every day!

4th phase: geroprotectors

The new stars of age research! Geroprotectors
can stopage-related cell / tissue damage and
sometimes reverse it.

What does intelligent prevention mean?

● Level 3 as basic care

● From the age of 40, additional level 4

Most diseases have a lead time of 20 to 30 years!

The scientific standard

1.Free from genetically modified organisms
2.Always the complete plant complex
3.Only the most effective ingredients
4.Standardized on active ingredients
5.Free from animal testing
6.100% toxin free
7.Free from questionable fillers and
auxiliaries, e.g. B. Magnesium stearate

Phytochemicals and geroprotectors

As already mentioned, the supply of vitamins, minerals and trace elements is very important.

In total, we need 47 vital micronutrients every day that interact with one another!

Our body works like a gigantic biochemical factory!

If only one substance is missing, our metabolism slows down and our performance is reduced.

In addition, the need for vital substances increases with stress, sport and with increasing age !

It is important that all active ingredients are contained in *a* product, because the micro-nutrients are dependent on each other in a very specific ratio.

Food supplements are age dependent.

The main problem of the **younger generation** is undersupply. They usually consume too much sugar, fat and salt through an unbalanced diet. Most of them lack antioxidants, vitamins, trace elements and minerals.

Aging is called oxidation. D eswegen we need a wide range of "rust-protection products" (anti-oxidants) .to verb-provement of V genaration with vital substances.

In **the middle of life** we are under special stress. Family, professional career and financial obligations drain the body's nerves and reserves of strength.

The vitality declines, the first metabolic diseases such as rheumatism, fat metabolism disorders, cardiovascular problems and the burn-out syndrome are spreading!

Then multivitamins, which are nerve tonic and intelligently support the vascular system, are very important.

Z for improvement of energy generation, to support the heart, brain and eye health are omega 3 fatty acids Need Beer t igt.

It makes sense to support the stem cells in cell cleaning, cell repair and energy generation.

From the age of 60 we need an adequate supply of nutrients. In addition, "intelligent" food supplements should degenerative s metabolism, and counter-Organver changes. Particular attention is paid to the mitochondria, the energy power plants of our cells.

As the metabolism slows down , the rising demand for E nergy-providing   nutrient   substances d to ramatisch.

So you realize that the older we get, the more important smart supplementation is. You can read more about the background to the changes that happen in our body as we get older in the chapter "Aging Intervention".

You can find more information at:

https://sisel.net/delphin66

If you are interested, arrange a non-binding consultation appointment with me - either by phone or email.

You are solely responsible for your health.

Strengthening the immune system

A strong immune system helps to fight off all kinds of pathogens such as viruses and bacteria. This is particularly important in these special times - Corona.

Sea algae are of particular importance.

Here I would like to quote a leading figure:

Dr. Bettina-Hees (Germany's number 1 algae expert):

"Due to their high fiber content, algae ensure **healthy digestion** and detoxification. They also supply all cells in our body with **energy** and minerals, vitamins, trace elements and amino acids!

The specific active ingredients are particularly important for our **immune system**.

They work as natural **killers** against **bacteria**, **viruses**, **fungi** and even **tumor cells**! "

Particularly effective is a Kombination, seaweed with fulvic, the molecules of life.

What Makes Fulvic Acids the Molecules of Life?

● Vitamins can only work if
  there are enough minerals

● Any deficiency in one or more
  minerals always ends in a metabolic
  disorder and thus illness

● Unfortunately, our digestive system can
  not asorbed most of the ingested minerals

The lack of fulv in acid n has meanwhile been recognized by many scientists as an extremely decisive factor for deficiencies in nutrients and thus an important cause of the resulting diseases.

In addition to water and oxygen FULV is o acid probably the most essential substance for our lives.

Aging intervention

Aging intervention is the achievement of the 21st century. These include: **cell cleaning, cell repair** and **cell rejuvenation.** All of this is already possible.

Why should we worry about it? We all want to get older - just not get OLD. Aging leads to the **accumulation of cellular damage** , which leads to **malfunction** of cells and tissues. In addition , aging leads to **loss**

of cell material , we gradually "crumble" . That sounds very tough now, but we can counteract this and optimize the aging process. The base is located in a guide life-balanced and healthy r diet, moderate exercise and healthy m, ie a US-rich n bed (7 - 8 hours).

All of this is not enough to counteract the aging process from the age of 40.

The **activation of our youth genes** as well as **intelligent cell repair and detoxification** are essential for healthy aging!

Prof. Dr. David Sinclair from Harvard Medical School is one of the **greatest experts** in **researching** and **slowing down the aging process.** What he i n its erschienenem in October 2019 book "The End of Aging - The revolutionary medicine of tomorrow" describes were there at that time already .

Have you stopped the question asked what the cells young and healthy get? I would like to answer your question below. They are healthy stem cells, reduction of cell waste, reduction of glyco-toxins, increase in the molecules of life, repair of DNA (genetic material), removal of heavy metals and the activation of our youth genes - sirtuins.

What are *sirtuins* ?

Sirtuins are enzymes that perform important tasks in our cells. When we activate the sirtuins in our cells, we stimulate the **metabolism** andconsiderablyimprove our **cell protection.** At the same time, **we slow down cell**

aging and thus the **aging** process. <u>Result</u> : We stay **fit, young** and **healthy longer** .

Resveratrol, as it **is in black grapes, i** st **effective** sirtuin activator. There are over **12,000 studies** at www.pubmed.gov

Die science deals in great detail with resveratrol. Congresses are held every year that deal with this active ingredient. Resveratrol has a positive effect on eye health, cancer, inflammation and degenerative diseases - and these are not all areas of action!

Resveratrol has a **positive** effect on our **eye health.** It has a positive influence on the restoration of the **retinal structure** and **blood flow**, which improves the **oxygen supply!** Resveratrol **protects** our sensitive **retinal cells** from cell death. Resveratrol can reduce **metabolic deposits** (drusen) in the retina.

Resveratrol charges the battery in our cells. Mitochondria are the energy suppliers / power

plants in our cells. The older we get, the more the function of our mitochondria is impaired. This leads to the gradual decrease of many health parameters in our body, e.g. .B .: cardiovascular diseases, brain functions, bone and eye diseases, cancer and many more. Resveratrol increases the number of mitochondria and improves or rejuvenates their function.

Resveratrol has a **positive** effecton our **brain functions.** Studies show that resveratrol is an effective natural agent to **maintain** the **memory** andthe **minds** may be the decrease with age.

Studies show an **improved blood flow** and **oxygen supply to** the brain as well as an **improved memory performance.**

Resveratrol has a **positive** effecton our **skin health.**

Resveratrol offers a powerful and scientifically based active ingredient that **rejuvenates** and **energizes** the skin.

According to studies, Resveratrol can help increase the **elasticity** and the **base moisture ness of the skin** to improve and above **oxidative S amage** to protect.

The first traces of the skin aging you can see from 30 the skin loses its elasticity and resilience. It becomes thinner and drier and the first wrinkles become visible!

How much and **which** *resveratrol* do we need?

Prof. Dr. David Sinclair:

" You would have to drink more than a hundred glasses of red wine every day to achieve the required effect!"

Resveratrol **is a mimosa.**

If the resveratrol molecule comes into contact with oxygen, it is destroyed!

The active ingredient is very poorly absorbed in form.

In the chapter on my holistic health concept, I had already written about Sisel International. This Science lab has developed a World Patent and used **patented nanotechnology** for the preparation of Eternity in **liquidr** form .

This increases bioavailability up to 250 times compared to resveratrol capsules.

It would **40 bottles of red wine** need **a r day serving Eternity** to match.

Among the **advantages n** of nanoverkapseltem resveratrol writes **Bill Sardi, a medical journalist, in his book "Anti-aging breakthrough":**

*" Can you imagine that **someone who takes resveratrol on a daily basis will** most likely live much **longer** and **healthier than others ? - That is remarkable ! "***

Next, I'll go into the topic of **stem cells** and regeneration.

Stem cells are used to form all cells, such as B. muscle cells, blood cells, nerve cells, etc. are required.

Stem cells contribute to the renewal and regeneration of organs and tissues.

However, with increasing age, the stem cells lose their function. By the age of **20** we have around **25 million** stem cells in our blood. At the age of **64** the stem cells have already reduced to around **5 million** .

Statement from science:

When the **aging mechanisms** of the tribe for economic **slowing**, we would allow a **longer** and **healthier** enabling lifet.

The functionality of the stem cells can be increased again through highly developed nutrients for the stem cells and support in reducing cell waste.

The next topic is the *reduction of glyco toxins.*

Glyco-toxins result from saccharification and are stubborn slagging. If sugar in our m oxidized body, they combine with protein and fatty acids to large macromolecules. They are called *glyco toxins* , as some of them are harmful to health!

Glyco-toxins area major cause of aging and the development of degenerative damage and diseases from the age of 35. Then more and more **age pigments** (lipofuscin) accumulate in our cells. This also affects the **brain** , **heart** , **liver** and **eyes** , whose function is impaired by the accumulation of **cell waste** .

When we are 40 years old, we already have 7 times as much cell waste lying around than when we were 10 years old.

The **cell division** is inhibited, thereby the tissue renewal slows, **allergies** be promoted and **detoxification** **processes** are weakened.

The **skin** loses its elasticity, as a result, is it thinner and more wrinkled. Age spots appear on the skin - the visible signs of cell waste. The **walls of the arteries** harden, which leads to circulatory disorders .

G lyko toxins are also visible in the eye lens. The clouding of the lens of the eye, which progresses with the aging process, leads to reduced visual acuity and to scattered light when driving at night. At an advanced stage, a cataract can develop.

Regular disposal of waste, i st as necessary as breathing! Glyco-toxins literally make us look old faster!

A final topic I would like to turn to the *molecules of life and the repair of DNA* .

NAD **+ is an important key to healthy aging!**

As we get older, the **NAD + level** in our

cells decreases . *NAD* + is a **key coenzyme** used by our mitochondria for **energy production** in all cells. A higher NAD + level is required so that our **cell communication** functions optimally. **The decrease in the NAD + level is one of the elementary biomarkers of aging!**

The older we get, the more cell damage increases! This ENORM increases the **health risk** .

Stress, environmental poisons / toxins and UV radiation v erstärken dramatically the number of cell damage.

That is why we need "**intelligent prevention**".

In a three-month self-experiment, Prof. Dr. David Sinclair found that NAD + can rejuvenate cells and thus even reverse the aging process. His biological age dropped from 57 years to 31.4 years (he was actually 47 years old).

" Prof. Dr. David Sinclair describes the

discovery as the greatest breakthrough since the
discovery of the antibiotic "

A crisis as an opportunity

With my holistic health concept, consisting of the components yoga, Qi Gong and Shiatsu already described, rounded off with my consultations on the subject of "healthy nutrition", I had realized my lifelong dream. For this I had given up my supposedly secure job as an office clerk and dared to venture into completely new and insecure territory. It's been a long road with many ups and downs.

After 10 years, I believed that I had set up my concept in such a way that I could make a living from it.

Then in March 2020 came the Corona crisis with its restrictions, which you, dear readers, are still familiar with.

Again I faced a new challenge. From now on, all

my appointments were canceled. I was wondering what's next? How do b I ekomme my earnings? Solutions had to be found. I had to reinvent myself.

I quickly got the intuition to offer one of my yoga classes online. I asked my participants if they wanted to try this experiment with me. Finally, I was once again breaking new ground. They were ready for it. Then I looked for a suitable platform and worked more and more into the technical possibilities. After just a few appointments, my participants enjoyed taking part in the yoga class from their living room so much that they longed to do it that way. You have saved time and travel, which is particularly advantageous in bad weather or in the dark. Since then, Tuesday evening has been reserved for the yoga class at 7 p.m.

After a few online appointments for the yoga class, I thought to myself: what works with yoga is also possible with Qi Gong. Thought - done. First, I tested out with a participant how Qi Gong felt in the online version. Finally I was alone in the room and the energetic vibration of the other group participants was missing. The usual energy field in the group could not be built up. Lo and behold - it felt good. Since I already had a few weeks of experience with my online yoga course, it made no difference to me whether I led the course alone in front of the camera or with the group in a room.

The other participants, who were otherwise in a group offer in Düsseldorf, were quickly won over for the online Qi Gong course. They also liked being able to take part in the course from their living room.

When the first easing occurred and courses could take place live again, I took advantage of the opportunities that were offered to me. This enabled me to win back my beloved participants.

With Qi Gong, too, those participants who were in the online course wanted to stay online rather than switch back to the live course.

The once established online courses (yoga and Qi Gong) were from then on part of my standard offer and I expanded them even further. A NEW idea was born!

The online services make t s me more flexible, because I no longer localized was . A new concept was born: to mix offline (on-site offers) with online offers.

Then it came to marketing and customer acquisition. I had arrived in the new, digital world!

A lot was offered digitally during the Corona crisis. This is how I became aware of a webinar on the subject of "video marketing" on a social network. I've always been interested in marketing - so I signed up. But video marketing? Well, another completely new area! The webinar was very interesting and I ordered the corresponding book to deepen it. I got deeper and deeper into the matter. Finally, I produced my own videos on yoga and Qi Gong. Then I created my own YouTube channel and uploaded the videos:

Yoga: https://www.youtube.com/playlist?list=PLGCBtDicniZxGuptIETMk1yHPpJUdk8eS

Qi Gong: https://www.youtube.com/playlist?list=PLGCBtDicniZwVdDDpk7R-apewddFLzmfQ

Since I also offer individual, holistic health concepts for individuals (personal training), this is also possible in Düsseldorf and online. I will adjust to your situation and see what you need right now. This can be exercises from yoga or Qi Gong or advice on all aspects of "healthy eating".

More videos were added later. I thought of the working people who want to do something for their health during their lunch break in the office or in the home office so that they can go back to work fit in the afternoon. The building blocks exercise, relaxation and nutrition also play a role.

Fit in the office:
https://www.youtube.com/playlist? list = PLGCBtDicniZyFwclUbdeEo14rHgAEoRkH

But that's not all! I used the time freed up by the crisis for other projects. So I can get the idea to create a blog. This also gave me a lot of pleasure and I was able to be creative again because it was again new territory. You can check out my blog at:

https://angelikadoerenberg.blogspot.com/

Find.

In order to round off my holistic health concepts, I decided to take up further training as a certified specialist advisor for

● Aging intervention

● Nutritional advice and

● Eye care

to be completed in the LongLife Academy.

It's an innovative healthcare home business based on 21st century nutritional science.

Since I was in the flow, I finally continued to write this book. I started it in September 2019. After a creative break of 9 months, during which I got pregnant with the subject of this book, it was completed during the Corona crisis. So this crisis changed my life in a positive way.

bibliography

● Kundalini, the secret of life
  by Swami Muktananda,
  Siddah Yoga Verlag GmbH,
  ISBN: 3-930711-28-1

● Atlas of Holistic Healing by
  Anna Elisabeth Röcker,
  Ludwig Verlag,
  ISBN: 3-7787-3699-X

● The Handbook of Chinese
  Medicine
  by Dr. Michael Grandjean and Dr.
  Klaus Birker,
  Joy-Verlag
  ISBN: 3-928554-19-0

● Licht & Liebe by Ursula Polaczek,
  self-published

- Kirtan - mantra singing,
  Yoga Vidya Verlag
  ISBN: 3-931854-22-1

- The three pillars of Qi Gong; Carsten
  Dohnke, Tao Hamburg

- The healing power of the mudras
  by Acharya Keshav Dev
  Via Nova Verlag
  ISBN: 3-936486-78-6

- Specialist lectures by Horst Altenfeld, LongLife
Academy

imprint

According to § 5 TMG:

Angelika Dörenberg
Institute Delphin
Roseggerstr. 12
40470 Düsseldorf

Contact:
Telephone: +49 (0) 211/6 41 62 85
Mobile: +49 (0)
152/21 64 83 64 E-Mail: info@institut-delphin.de

www.ingramcontent.com/pod-product-compliance
Lightning Source LLC
Chambersburg PA
CBHW031235250726
48655CB00005B/1967